VEGAN DIET

30 All Time Classic Vegan Recipes, Everything from Breakfast to Dessert

(Easy and Healthy Vegan Diet Recipes That Will Make You Feel Better)

Chris Ford

Published by Robert Satterfield Publishing House

© **Chris Ford**

All Rights Reserved

Vegan Diet: 30 All Time Classic Vegan Recipes, Everything from Breakfast to Dessert (Easy and Healthy Vegan Diet Recipes That Will Make You Feel Better)

ISBN 978-1-989682-96-8

All rights reserved. No part of this guide may be reproduced in any form without permission in writing from the publisher except in the case of brief quotations embodied in critical articles or reviews.

Legal & Disclaimer

The information contained in this book is not designed to replace or take the place of any form of medicine or professional medical advice. The information in this book has been provided for educational and entertainment purposes only.

The information contained in this book has been compiled from sources deemed reliable, and it is accurate to the best of the Author's knowledge; however, the Author cannot guarantee its accuracy and validity and cannot be held liable for any errors or omissions. Changes are periodically made to this book. You must consult your doctor or get professional medical advice before using any of the suggested remedies, techniques, or information in this book.

TABLE OF CONTENT

PART 1 1

INTRODUCTION 2

CHAPTER 1: PLANT-BASED SUPERFOODS FOR OPTIMAL HEALTH 4

What are Superfoods? 4
Plant-Based Superfoods 5
List of Plant-based Superfoods 6

CHAPTER 2: BENEFITS OF PLANT-BASED SUPERFOOD DIET 16

Increased Energy and Muscle Gain 20
Reduced Inflammation and Body Acidity 23

CHAPTER 3: VEGETARIAN SUPERFOOD RECIPES 30

AVOCADO-COCONUT MATCHA SMOOTHIE 30

CACAO BLUEBERRY-KEFIR SMOOTHIE 31

MIXED BERRY SPIRULINA SMOOTHIE 32

SUPERFOOD GRANOLA BARS 33

MIXED SEEDS CRISP BREADS 35

OATMEAL CACAO BREAKFAST BAR 37

WILD RICE BREAKFAST PUDDING 40

BREAKFAST SPROUTED GRAIN SALAD 42

SHREDDED COCONUT QUINOA-CHIA PORRIDGE 43

SUPERFOOD BREAKFAST ACAI BOWL 45

10 SUPERFOOD VEGETARIAN MAIN DISH RECIPES	47
ROASTED VEGETABLES AND MARINATED HEMP FU	47
CREAMY NAVY BEAN SOUP WITH WILD RICE	49
BROCCOLI AND FAVA SALAD	51
SPICY GRILLED HEMP FU WITH MIXED BEAN SALAD	53
EDAMAME-QUINOA KALE SALAD	56
FAVA GREEN SALAD WITH QUINOA AND AVOCADO SAUCE	58
AVOCADO BULGUR GREEN SALAD WITH FRIED HEMP FU	60
ARUGULA AND FAVA SALAD WITH APRICOTS AND HEMP FU	62
CURRIED BULGUR AND LIMA BEANS WITH SQUASH	64
FAVA AND BROCCOLI SALAD WITH TAHINI DRESSING	67
CONCLUSION	69
PART 2	71
INTRODUCTION	72
CHAPTER 1: A BRIEF VEGAN HISTORY	73
CHAPTER 2: THE CENTRAL DIET FOR VEGANS	85
CHAPTER 3: STARTER RECIPES	98
STIR FRIED TOFU WITH BROCCOLI	100
CHAPTER 4: FOOD GROUPS	104
CHAPTER 5: COLORS OF THE FARM	112
CHAPTER 6: TASTING THE NUTRITION	114

CHAPTER 7: WEIGHT LOSS AND DIETS	**117**
CONCLUSION	**126**
ABOUT THE AUTHOR	**127**

Part 1

Introduction

The Vegan Haven provides detailed information on how a Vegetarian diet provides a complete and balanced nutrition to meet the body's nutritional needs. It also contains the best sources of plant-based foods from all major food groups to supply the body with right amounts and types of nutrients that are essential in maintaining optimal health and for proper functioning of the body.

Within this book, we will be talking about the benefits of doing a Vegetarian diet with emphasis on nutrient-dense foods from plant-based sources that are known to possess beneficial and medicinal properties. These nutrient-dense foods are termed as "SUPERFOODS". Superfoods have long been recognized for their anti-aging and immune-boosting properties that can contribute in healthy aging and longevity. Other benefits of eating plant-based superfoods include prevention and treatment of certain health diseases, reduced cardiovascular risks, controlled blood sugar and cholesterol, higher levels of energy, healthy weight loss, body mass regulation, enhanced digestive health, increased nutrient absorption, improved health status and successful aging.

With a plant-based superfood diet, optimum health is achieved and risks to various health disease and conditions are effectively reduced. There is no specific form of diet that has been scientifically proven and tested in humans that can directly influence or increase longevity. But with regular consumption of nutrient-dense foods like plant-based superfoods, a well-nourished body is maintained, and also kept healthy, strong and disease-free to promote successful aging and longevity.

In this book, you can find healthy and delicious vegetarian superfood recipes that easy to prepare and are specially created to provide you with varied and tasty vegetarian recipes. Try these flavorful vegetarian recipes now to supply your body with beneficial nutrients for a stronger immune system, higher levels of energy and promote overall health and increase longevity.

Chapter 1: Plant-Based Superfoods for Optimal Health

What are Superfoods?

Plant-based superfoods are packed with nutrients and antioxidants making it the best foods for a healthy balanced diet. Superfoods contain all essential nutrients that the body requires including vitamins, minerals, healthy fats, dietary fiber and proteins. They are also rich in beneficial and medicinal substances such as antioxidants, anti-cancer and anti-inflammatory compounds.

Various health and healing benefits are acquired when superfoods are integrated in vegetarian diet, including healthy weight loss, muscle gain, increased energy, stronger immune system, improved digestive health, regulated sugar and cholesterol levels, healthy aging and enhanced longevity.

It is also the healthiest form of diet because it recommends consuming mainly on foods that provide sufficient levels of nutrients to meet the body's nutritional requirements and to gain optimum health.

Majority of the plant-based superfoods are basically low in calories and free from harmful substances making it the best sources of foods for longevity.

Plant-Based Superfoods

One of your most basic health principles is to eat a diet of whole, nutritious foods rather than processed types in order maintain a healthy weight and improve overall health. Feeding your body the right nutrients rather than stuffing it with "empty" calories will not only help you lose unwanted pounds, it's a key ingredient for living a long and healthy life. Believe it or not, many people who are obese are actually profoundly malnourished.

The Best Sources of Superfoods:

· Readily available and unprocessed or unrefined

· Rich in nutrients are known to promote longevity

- Provides health benefits that are supported with research and studies or scientifically proven

List of Plant-based Superfoods

Cacao

Raw cacao is a healthy source of fats and rich in antioxidants that are higher or equivalent with other widely known sources such as acai berries and blueberries, pomegranate and other fruits. The types of antioxidants from cacao help protect against heart-related diseases, promote cardiovascular health, and promotes normal functioning of the nervous system.

It is recommended to consume raw cacao and unsweetened cacao nibs.

Berries

Acai Berries

Acai berries are packed with essential fatty acids, amino acids and antioxidants. The beneficial properties of acai berries include increased energy, regulated cholesterol levels, improved digestive health, and enhanced overall health and well-being.

Goji Berries

Goji berries contain high amounts of vitamin A, vitamin C, Vitamin B12, iron, selenium and antioxidants. These nutrients can help boost the immune system, fight against cancer, prevent cardiovascular diseases, and enhance brain functioning to increase lifespan.

Blueberries

Blueberries are rich in antioxidants that can help improve brain and nerve functioning, reduce age-related disease and conditions, eliminate free radicals and toxins, enhance digestion and reduce inflammation.

Other Superfood Fruits:

- Noni Berries

- *Cherries*

- *Pomegranate*

- *Mangosteen*

- *Blackberries*
- *Gooseberries*
- Bilberries

Seaweeds and Algae

Seaweeds and sea vegetables are excellent sources of dietary protein, rich in minerals (calcium, iodine, iron and magnesium) and high in vitamin C.

The natural iodine contained from these foods is essential in maintaining a functional thyroid gland. It also has antibacterial, anti-inflammatory and anti-viral properties and health benefits including prevention of cardiovascular diseases and diabetes, regulates blood sugar levels, improved memory, better eyesight and enhanced functioning of the liver.

Spirulina

Spirulina is a type of micro-algae that is one of the many superfoods and is considered as a complete food because it contains ample amounts of essential macronutrients, micronutrients and other beneficial compounds needed by the body.

Health benefits of adding spirulina into the diet include damage and repair of damaged cells, increased energy, fights aging and maintenance of overall health.

Chlorella

Chlorella, a blue-green algae that is related with spirulina is a great natural source of essential amino acids, beta-carotene, chlorophyll, potassium, magnesium, phosphorous, biotin and B-complex vitamins. It contains high levels and many types of beneficial compounds that can help increase energy, boost the immune system, fight against cancer, regulate blood sugar and cholesterol levels, promote weight loss and eliminate toxic metals, free radicals and radioactive particles in the body.

Cruciferous Vegetables

Cruciferous vegetables have amazing nutritional and healing properties that help to enhance proper functioning of different systems in the body including detoxification of harmful chemicals and toxins, enhanced digestive health and complete food digestion and nutrient absorption, facilitates weight loss due to ample amounts of fiber, and promotes overall health by giving the body with essential vitamins and minerals.

Cruciferous vegetables are basically high in anti-cancer compounds together with, dietary fiber, minerals, vitamins, protein, natural fatty acids and potent antioxidants. These vegetables provide healing properties and health benefits including cancer prevention, reduced cardiovascular risks, healthy aging, regulated blood glucose and cholesterol levels, improved digestive health and maintenance of estrogen levels.

List of Cruciferous Vegetables:

· *Broccoli*

· Cauliflower

· *Cabbage*

- Brussels Sprouts

- *Turnips*

- *Radish*

- **Horseradish**

Leafy Greens

Green leafy vegetables are great sources of dietary fiber and known to have several anticancer properties. This group of vegetables includes spinach, kale, bok choy and pak choy, collard and turnip greens and nettle.

Nettle

Nettle contains high amounts and excellent sources of plant protein, chlorophyll and essential vitamins including Vitamins A, C and D. Health benefits include enhanced thyroid function, increase body metabolism and better digestion. It is also beneficial during pregnancy, helps in blood clotting and improves kidney function.

Spinach

Spinach is an excellent source of iron, Vitamins A, C, E and K, and is rich in minerals including B-complex, folic acid, fatty acids, calcium, potassium, protein, phosphorus, zinc, selenium and omega-3 fatty acids.

Spinach is also rich in dietary fiber, folic acid and antioxidants that are proven effective in the elimination of body wastes and toxic metals, enhance food digestion, improve digestive health and increase nutrient absorption.

Other leafy greens include:

• *Kale*

• Romaine and Leaf Lettuce

• Mustard and Collard Greens

• Chicory and Swiss Chard

Nuts, Seeds, Grains and Beans

The nutrients and compounds from nuts have been linked with reduced cardiovascular risks. Almonds are not only healthy sources of proteins and fats, but are also rich in antioxidants that are known to maintain a healthy heart. Peanuts are rich in anti-cancer compounds or flavonoids, known as resveratrol. Walnuts and Brazil nuts are healthy sources of selenium which have been proven to help prevent heart-related diseases and cancer. Nuts can also help in regulating glucose and insulin levels that can influence in treating Type 2 Diabetes.

Raw Macadamia Nuts

Contains essential nutrients including dietary protein and ample amounts of monounsaturated fat that helps reduce cholesterol levels, reduce cardiovascular risks, healthy weight loss, and speeds up body metabolism.

Hemp Seeds

Is a healthy source of protein, omega-3 and omega-6 that are proven to help in maintaining a healthy heart, regulating blood pressure and cholesterol levels.

Chia Seeds

Chia seeds are rich in dietary protein, essential fatty acids and soluble fiber. These nutrients are the basic requirements to promote weight loss.

Quinoa and Amaranth

Quinoa and amaranth are healthy sources of natural protein, manganese, magnesium, fiber, copper and other compounds that are contained in high amounts to meet the body's nutritional needs.

Buckwheat

Buckwheat is rich in phytonutrients that are known to protect against breast cancers and other types of cancers that are hormone-dependent.

Plant-Based Sources of Fats

Coconut Oil

Coconut oil is considered as one of the best superfoods for longevity. It is also a healthy source of dietary fat because it is easier to digest compared to the others. And since be converted quickly into energy instead of storing it in the body as fat. It also naturally slows aging by lowering oxidative stress. Prevents heart diseases and high blood pressure it helps convert the "bad" or LDL cholesterols into good cholesterols. A

Avocado oil

Avocados are excellent sources of monounsaturated fat which is proven to aid in burning fats, increasing energy levels and weight loss.

Flaxseed oil

Flaxseed oil contains a type of fat known as alpha-linolenic acid which helps reduce blood cholesterol levels and prevent heart-related problems. It has also been known to enhance kidney function.

Fermented Vegetables

These superfoods are rich in probiotics which are beneficial in maintaining a healthy gut, enhancing digestive health and increasing absorption of nutrients from digested foods. They also contain high amounts of antioxidants that are needed in eliminating toxic metals and free radicals in the body.

Chapter 2: Benefits of Plant-based Superfood Diet

Improved Digestive Health and Enhance

Nutrient Absorption
It is very important to maintain a healthy and functional digestive system in order to properly digest foods, avoid gut problems related with incomplete digestion of foods and increase the amount of nutrients that are absorbed by the body. By following the Vegetarian diet, it can enhance digestion and promote efficient functioning of the digestive system, thus increasing nutrient absorption from plant-based foods and improving overall health.

When digestive health is neglected, certain conditions are acquired by the body including inflammations of the gut villi, digestive tract infections and damages in the intestinal linings. These digestive problems occur when foods are not properly digested or contain substances that can trigger auto-immune conditions or allergies. Damaged and inflamed gut linings are incapable of fully digesting certain foods and inefficient in absorbing the nutrients given by the foods we eat. If left untreated, it can complicate to serious health problems and diseases such as malnutrition or nutrient deficiencies, stomach ulcers and certain cancers of digestive organs.

In order to keep a healthy and functional digestive system and to improve nutritional status, it is suggested to consume more on nutrient-dense plant-based foods that are free of harmful substances and can trigger auto-immune disorders. Integrate superfoods with Vegetarian diet to have sufficient levels of nutrients to meet the body's nutritional requirement, and in order to maintain a strong immune system, prevent health problems and diseases and to improve overall health for increased longevity.

Healthy Weight Loss and Burning of Stored Body Fats

With a plant-based superfood diet, reducing body weight is made easy and burning of stored body fats are made effective. Plant-based foods are also excellent sources macronutrients including protein, fats and fiber which are satiating. Foods with high satiety values are very filling and can make you feel full for long durations, thus reducing appetite and food cravings and decreasing the amount of foods you eat.

Vegetarian diet can also help in burning the fats that are stored in the body due to excessive consumption of empty carbohydrates and sugar. High carbohydrate and sugar intake causes the body to rely on energy sources obtained from glucose metabolization. If energy sources from glucose are not spent, these are stored in the body as fats which are hard to remove or burn causing rapid gain in weight, obesity, diabetes, cardiovascular diseases.

When you eat foods that are high in protein, healthy sources of fats and fiber, it causes the body to metabolize fats that are stored in the body. It is also recommended to avoid foods with empty carbohydrates and processed sugars, so that the body effectively burn the body fats and convert them into energy as fuel sources. In addition, avoiding empty carbs and refined sugars can also help in regulating glucose levels. High levels of glucose in the blood can cause secretion of insulin rapidly which has been linked in gaining body weight, obesity, cardiovascular diseases and diabetes.

Vegetarian diet with emphasis on superfoods facilitates effective burning of body fats through increased protein and fat consumption with low carbohydrate diet. It is recommended to reduce the dietary intake of foods with high carbohydrate contents to avoid glucose metabolization as fuel source for the cell and brain. Reducing carbohydrate intake from unhealthy sources avoids various health diseases and problems such as obesity, Diabetes and heart related problems.

Increased Energy and Muscle Gain

Increased Energy Levels

Vegetarian diet with focus on superfoods can help increase energy levels and reduce the energy usage especially in digesting foods. The most energy-consuming bodily process is digestion that is why it is recommended to eat mainly on foods that are unprocessed, raw or from natural sources because these are easily digested and absorbed in the body. Plant-based superfoods are digested easily in the body, while processed and refined foods require lots of energy for the body to fully digest them. It is better to spend energy for other important functional purposes like building muscles, restorations and treatments of damaged organs in the body.

Unhealthy dieting has a direct relation with stress levels in the body. It has been proven that eating unhealthy foods or unhealthy eating habits can only increase stress levels in the body. Increased stress levels the body is also associated with various health problems including insomnia.

Superfoods and other plant-based foods contain natural enzymes if eaten fresh or raw. Raw and fresh foods can also be easily digested and absorbed in the body. With this, digestion is made easier and efficient, decreasing energy consumption and reducing stress levels acquired by unhealthy dieting. Since the diet keeps stress levels low or reduced, sleeping patterns is improved and developing insomnia is avoided thus increasing energy. And because the diet promotes burning body fats which converts them into energy, the body is given with extra sources of energy thus increasing the levels of energy.

Plant-based superfoods like almonds, cashews and hazelnuts are rich in magnesium which is an important mineral in converting nutrients into energy. Fermented vegetables like sauerkraut and kimchi are also considered as superfoods because of the probiotics present in these types of foods. The probiotics from fermented vegetables can help promote complete food digestion and increase the amount of nutrients absorbed into the body.

Muscle Growth and Recovery

Plant-based foods are among the best sources of protein which contain different types and high amounts of necessary amino acids. This type of nutrient is very important especially in repairing damaged muscle tissues and muscle growth. This process of replacing or repairing muscle tissues requires amino acids that are usually gained from protein-rich foods. Damage repair and muscle growth involve the process known as protein synthesis. Amino acids are essential in stimulating growth of leaner and stronger muscles, helps produce more energy, promotes bone strength and aids in collagen production.

Reduced Inflammation and Body Acidity

Inflammations are protective reactions made by the human body, specifically in the tissues caused by irritation, infection or injury that is characterized by redness, swelling, pain and sometimes loss of function. It is part of the body's immune response and without it, the body can't heal. These are reactions from food allergies, intestinal issues and other autoimmune diseases caused by consumption of various foods such as grains, legumes and dairy products. Inflammation is a serious problem that can lead to obesity and other health diseases, if left untreated. Avoiding foods that are processed and contain substances that cause inflammations in the body, and replacing them with whole organic foods will automatically reduce inflammations and restore gut health promoting an improved overall health.

Vegetarian diet provides food choices that can help reduce and treat inflammations. Dark leafy vegetables such as collard greens, spinach, kale and Swiss chard contain powerful and beneficial antioxidants, flavonoids, carotenoids, and vitamin C which help protect against cellular damage. Blueberries and other varieties contain high amounts of antioxidants essential in body detoxification reducing inflammatory reactions. Herbs and spices such as garlic, turmeric, ginger, parsley and pepper all contain anti-inflammatory elements.

It is important that the body maintains a balance of acidity and alkalinity. Imbalance between these two components leads to several health diseases like, osteoporosis, hypertension, asthma, insomnia and formation of kidney stones. Plant-based superfood provides a neutral effect when eaten regularly, which means the acidity level is balanced with the alkalinity of foods. Grains, dairy products like hard cheeses and salty processed foods produce a net acid load after digestion and cause health problems and diseases. Since Vegetarian diet recommends in eating protein rich foods together with many vegetables and adequate fruits, the net acid load is slightly alkaline thus reducing the risks of digestive problems and various health diseases caused by acidic body.

Immune System Strengthening, Body Detox and Anti-Aging

Plant based, nutrient-dense vegetables and fruits, especially superfoods provide many healing and anti-inflammatory benefits and can strengthen the immune system. Superfoods are basically rich in antioxidants which are essential in eliminating toxins and free radicals, and vital in speeding up your metabolism.

Herbs and spices such as garlic, red bell peppers, ginger and onions are proven to be effective in boosting the immune system. Ginger aids in proper food digestion for increased nutrient absorption, has anti-inflammatory elements that reduces pain. Plant-based superfoods are immune system enhancers because it contain high amounts of vitamin A and E, omega-3 fatty acids, beta-carotene, antioxidants and zinc which is very important for the development of white blood cells which destroys invading bacteria and viruses. Coconut products contain lauric acid which can help strengthen a person's immunity.

Another way of boosting the immune system is consuming more superfoods that are plant-based. It provides the needed nutrition to fight against aging like initiating probiotic growth, improving skin quality and removing wrinkles. Other anti-aging properties of the diet includes faster healing of wounds and improved immune body system functioning. High amount of antioxidants from superfoods are also essential in eliminating toxic chemicals, minerals and free radicals and keeping the liver healthy and restoring normal functioning of blood cells for effective blood circulation.

Regulated Cholesterol and Sugar Levels
Vegetarian diet promotes a steady, slow rise in the blood sugar and insulin levels through reducing carbohydrate and sugar consumption. Foods rich in sugar and empty carbs causes rapid rise of blood sugar and insulin levels which is the

primary cause of obesity, hypertension, unhealthy blood lipid and cholesterol levels, and Type 2 diabetes.

Blood levels of the hormone insulin lower down when consumption of carbohydrate is reduced. High insulin level contributes to fat storage and low insulin level facilitates fat burning, a result of high protein and low carb diet. Maintaining steady level of blood sugar is very important because our body breaks these foods easily which can cause abrupt elevation of blood sugar level that can lead to various health problems and diseases. The Vegetarian diet eliminates or reduces food groups that alter the blood sugar levels too much like grains and foods rich in sugar and suggests in eating primarily on vegetables and fruits sources to help stabilize blood sugar levels.

Successful Aging and Longevity

Healthy aging is not only described as the absence of diseases and conditions associated with aging, but identified as maintenance and development of optimal social, physical and mental proper functioning and well-being. Vegetarian diet has shown significant results in improving overall health that can help promote longevity and successful aging.

By following the Vegetarian diet, healthy aging can be achieved by preventing and reducing the risks to age-related health diseases and conditions, and by restoring health for proper functioning of all systems in the body. Vegetarian diet has shown significant results like anti-aging benefits and provided positive effects to health including better sleep, higher levels of energy, healthy weight loss and in burning stored body fats. It can also help improve immune health, reduce chronic inflammatory pain and diseases, and reduce the risk of cardiovascular disease and other health changes in promoting overall health and longevity for successful aging. Plant-based superfoods also provide beneficial nutrients essential in making new healthy cells and in strengthening the immune system. The majority of plant-based foods are rich in antioxidants, vitamins and minerals that can help eliminate toxins and free radicals and prevent early aging and development of age-related conditions such as heart-related problems and diseases, diabetes, joint inflammations and bone diseases. Foods groups that are restricted in the Vegetarian diet such as animal meat and by products, processed foods, dairy products and refined oils and sugars contain elements that can greatly affect in the development of age-related conditions and diseases and affect health and lifespan.

Chapter 3: Vegetarian Superfood Recipes

10 Superfood Vegetarian Breakfast Recipes

Avocado-Coconut Matcha Smoothie

Preparation Time: 5 minutes

Serves: 2

Ingredients:

- 1 teaspoon matcha powder
- ½ cup coconut cream
- 1 cup almond milk
- 1 large avocado, pitted
- 1 scoop vegan vanilla protein powder
- 1 tablespoon of raw honey (optional)
- 2 cubes of coconut water (optional)

Directions:

1. Combine all ingredients in a high speed blender or food processor and pulse for about 30 seconds on medium-low speed.

Turn to high speed and pulse until thick and smooth.

2. Divide into two serving glasses and serve immediately.

Cacao Blueberry-Kefir Smoothie

Preparation Time: 5 minutes

Serves: 2

Ingredients:

- 1 cup of organic vanilla kefir
- ½ cup plain soy yogurt
- 1 cup of frozen blueberries
- 2 tablespoons of raw cacao powder
- 1 small pinch of cinnamon
- 1 tablespoon of pure maple syrup

For the Topping:
- ½ teaspoon of cacao nibs, for topping
- 1 tablespoon of bee pollen, for topping

Directions:

1. Mix all ingredients in a food processor or high speed blender and pulse for about 30 seconds on medium-low speed. Adjust to high speed and pulse until thick and smooth.

2. Transfer into two serving glasses, top with cacao nibs and bee pollen and serve immediately.

Mixed Berry Spirulina Smoothie

Preparation Time: 5 minutes

Serves: 2

Ingredients:

- 1 1 ½ teaspoons of spirulina
- ½ cup of kefir or soy yogurt
- 1 cup of soy milk
- 1 cup of frozen blueberries
- ½ cup of frozen raspberries
- 2 tablespoons of dried Goji berries

- Chia seeds or shredded coconut flakes, for topping (optional)

Directions:

1. Add all ingredients in a high speed blender or food processor and pulse for about 30 seconds on medium-low speed. Turn to high speed and pulse until thick and smooth.

2. Transfer into two serving glasses and top with chia seeds and shredded coconut flakes, if desired. Serve immediately.

Superfood Granola Bars

Preparation Time: 5 minutes

Cooking Time: 30 minutes

Serves: 8 to 12

Ingredients:

- 1 cup of almond meal

- ½ cup of mixed seeds

- 2 tablespoons of hemp seeds

- 1 ½ cups of old fashioned oats
- ½ cup of ground old fashioned oats
- ½ cup of dried goji berries
- ½ cup raw cacao nibs
- 2 tablespoons of Maca powder
- 1 teaspoon of ground cinnamon
- ¼ cup of raw honey
- ¼ cup of pure maple syrup
- 3 to 4 tablespoons of melted coconut oil

Directions:

1. Preheat the oven to 350°F, line a baking dish (8x8) with foil and lightly grease with oil. Set aside.

2. Mix all dry ingredients in a large mixing bowl.

3. Melt the coconut oil in a saucepan, remove the saucepan from heat and stir in the honey and maple syrup. Whisk until

well combined and add into the dry mixture.

4. Mix it thoroughly until all of the ingredients are well incorporated. Transfer into the prepared baking dish and press it down until uniformly packed on all sides.

5. Bake it in the oven for about 30 minutes, or until the edges are golden brown. Remove from the oven, transfer to a wire rack and let it rest to cool completely. Turn unto a cutting board and cut into squares.

6. Serve immediately, or place it inside airtight container and store it in the fridge for future consumption.

Mixed Seeds Crisp breads

Preparation Time: 5 minutes

Cooking Time: 25 minutes

Serves: 6 to 8

Ingredients:
- ½ cup of mixed seeds

- 2 tablespoons of flax seeds

- ¼ cup chia seeds

- ¼ cup of old fashioned oats

- ¼ cup of stone-ground flour

- ½ teaspoon of pink Himalayan salt or real salt

- 1 cup of coconut water or filtered

- ¼ cup of raw honey or 2 tablespoons of agave nectar

- 2 tablespoons of melted coconut oil

Directions:

1. Preheat the oven to 300°F.

2. Place the honey and coconut water in a small bowl, whisk until well combined and set aside.

3. In a separate mixing bowl, combine all dry ingredients and stir in the oil and honey mixture. Mix it thoroughly until well combined, cover then bowl and let it stand for 30 minutes.

4. Prepare two sheets of parchment paper while the mixture is resting. Transfer the mixture on top of one parchment paper. Cover with remaining parchment paper and roll out the mixture into very thin sheet.

5. Remove the parchment paper on top. Slice into squares but do not separate it yet and transfer to a baking sheet. Bake it in the oven for about 25 minutes, or until crisp and lightly golden.

6. Remove from the oven, transfer to a wire rack and let it rest to cool before breaking into squares. Serve immediately or store it in airtight containers.

Oatmeal Cacao Breakfast Bar

Preparation Time: 10 minutes

Cooking Time: 25 minutes

Serves: 16

Ingredients:

For the Base:
- 2 cups stone-ground oats

- 1 cup of sliced or slivered almonds
- 2 tablespoons of cacao nibs
- 1 teaspoon Celtic sea salt
- ½ tablespoon of ground cinnamon
- 2 medium ripe bananas, diced
- 1 scoop of vegan protein powder
- 1 teaspoon of pure vanilla extract
- 2 to 3 teaspoons of coconut oil
- ¼ cup of raw honey

For the Top Layer:
- ½ cup of rolled oats
- ¼ cup of sliced almonds
- 2 tablespoons of chia seeds
- 2 tablespoons of hemp seeds
- 1 cup of fresh blueberries
- ¼ cup of almond or soy milk (or plain coconut or plain almond milk)

- 1 large pinch of ground cinnamon
- 1 teaspoon of raw cacao powder

Directions:

1. Preheat the oven to 350°F, line a baking pan (9x9) with parchment paper and lightly grease with oil. Set aside.

2. In a large mixing bowl, add all dry ingredients for the base and stir in the wet ingredients. Mix until well incorporated and transfer into the prepared baking pan. Press it down to fill the empty spaces in the baking pan and spread evenly to have uniform thickness. Bake it in the oven for 10 minutes, transfer to a wire rack and let it rest while preparing the mixture for the top layer.

3. While baking the base, combine all ingredients for the top layer and add it into the base. Spread it evenly on top of the base and press down to fill empty spaces. Bake it for another 15 minutes or the mixture has set.

4. Remove from the oven, transfer to a wire rack and let it rest to cool completely. Cut into squares and store it in airtight containers.

Wild Rice Breakfast Pudding

Preparation Time: 10 minutes

Cooking Time: 35 minutes

Serves: 4

Ingredients:

• 1 cup fresh blueberries

• 1 cup quartered fresh strawberries

• 1 ripe banana, peeled and sliced

• 1 teaspoon of ground cinnamon, for topping

• 1 tablespoon of shredded coconut flakes, for topping

For the Yogurt Mixture:
• 2 cups kefir or soy yogurt

- 2 tablespoons of maple syrup or raw honey, or as needed to taste

- 2 tablespoons of sprouted chia seeds

- ¼ cup of soy or hemp milk

For the Wild Rice:
- 1 cup of wild rice, rinsed and drained

- 1 cup of water

- 1 cup of unsweetened almond or coconut milk

Directions:

1. Place all ingredients for the yogurt mixture, briefly stir to combine and let it stand while preparing the other ingredients for the chia seeds to sprout.

2. Rinse the wild rice under cool running water until the drained water runs clear. Simmer it in a pan with salted boiling water for 30 to 35 minutes, or until tender. Remove from heat and set aside until the rice has fully absorbed the liquid.

3. In a large mixing bowl, add in the blueberries, strawberries, banana, wild rice and yogurt mixture and gently toss to combine.

4. Divide into 4 serving bowls and sprinkle with cinnamon and coconut flakes on top. Serve immediately or chill before serving.

Breakfast Sprouted Grain Salad

Preparation Time: 5 minutes

Cooking Time: N/A

Serves: 6 to 8

Ingredients:

- 2 cups of sprouted rolled oats

- 1 cup sprouted quinoa

- ½ cup sprouted millet

- 1 cup soy yogurt or kefir

- ½ cup of vanilla hemp or almond milk

- 1 large pinch of nutmeg

- ½ teaspoon of ground ginger

- ½ cup of sliced almonds
- ½ cup of dry-roasted cashews
- 1 cup of fresh blueberries or strawberries

For the Honey Lime Dressing:
- ¼ cup of coconut oil or flax oil
- 2 organic limes, juiced and zested
- ½ cup of raw honey or maple syrup

Directions:

1. In a large mixing bowl, add the sprouted oats, quinoa, cashew, almond and blueberries. Pour in the soy yogurt and hemp milk and season to taste with ginger powder and nutmeg. Gently toss to combine and divide into four serving bowls.

2. Drizzle with honey lime dressing and serve immediately.

Shredded Coconut Quinoa-Chia Porridge
Preparation Time: 10 minutes

Cooking Time: 10 minutes

Serves: 6 to 8

Ingredients:

- 2 cups of sprouted quinoa (soaked and drained)
- 1 cup of sprouted chia seeds
- ½ cup dried Goji berries
- 1 cup of shredded coconut flakes
- 1 cup of plain soy or almond milk
- ½ cup of soy yogurt
- ½ teaspoon of ground cinnamon
- 3 to 4 tablespoons of pure maple syrup or raw honey
- ¼ cup of chopped almonds
- 2 tablespoons of fresh bee pollen, for topping
- 2 tablespoons of extra shredded coconut, of topping

Directions:

1. Place the quinoa, chia seeds, Goji berries, coconut flakes, cinnamon, soy milk and yogurt in a large mixing bowl and briefly stir to combine. Cover the bowl and chill for at least 2 to 4 hours.

2. Remove from the chiller, transfer to a pan and stir in the almonds and maple syrup or honey. Cook until it reaches to a boil, or until warmed through.

3. Divide into four serving bowls and top with bee pollen and shredded coconut before serving.

Superfood Breakfast Acai Bowl

Preparation Time: 10 minutes

Cooking Time: N/A

Serves: 6 to 8

Ingredients:

For the Acai Mixture:
· 1 pack of unsweetened frozen acai puree, thawed and broken into pieces

· 1 ½ cups frozen blueberries

- 1 ½ cups sliced frozen bananas
- 1 ½ cups of almond or coconut milk
- 1 teaspoon of pure vanilla extract
- 1 scoop of vegan protein powder
- 2 tablespoons of raw honey or agave nectar

For the Toppings:
- 1 tablespoon of teaspoon cacao nibs
- 2 tablespoons of dried mixed seeds
- 2 tablespoons of dried mixed berries

Directions:

1. Place all ingredients for the acai mixture in a high speed blender or food processor, and pulse until thick and smooth.

2. Divide into four serving bowls, add with topping ingredients and serve immediately.

10 Superfood Vegetarian Main Dish Recipes

Roasted Vegetables and Marinated Hemp Fu

Preparation time: 20 minutes

Cooking time: 40 minutes

Serves: 3 to 4

Ingredients:

· 12 oz. of drained and pressed hemp Fu or soy tofu, cut into large cubes

· 1 large red sweet pepper, sliced into strips

· 1 cup of detached cauliflower florets

· 1 cup asparagus spears

· Real salt and black pepper, to taste

For the Marinade:
· 1/3 cup raw coconut aminos or namu shoyu

· 1 large organic lemon, juiced and zested

- 2 tablespoons of balsamic vinegar
- 2 tablespoons of raw honey
- 2 tablespoons of melted coconut oil
- 1 ½ teaspoons of minced garlic
- 1 small red onion, minced
- 1 teaspoon of turmeric powder
- 1 teaspoon of Italian seasoning mix

Directions:

1. Mix all marinade ingredients in a large non-reactive bowl, add in the tofu and gently toss to evenly coat with the marinade. Cover bowl and chill for at least 2 hours to marinate the tofu.

2. Preheat the oven to 380ºF, line two rimmed baking sheets with foil and set aside.

3. When the tofu is ready, drain and transfer into the prepared baking sheet.

4. Add the vegetables into the marinade mixture and gently toss to coat evenly.

Transfer into a separate prepared baking sheet and bake together with the hemp or soy tofu for 15 minutes in the oven.

5. Turn tofu and vegetables and bake further for about 15 to 20 minutes. Remove from the oven when the tofu is thoroughly cooked and the vegetables are tender.

6. Portion the vegetables into individual serving plates, top with tofu and serve immediately.

Creamy Navy Bean Soup with Wild Rice

Preparation time: 10 minutes

Cooking time: 50 to 60 minutes

Serves: 4 to 6

Ingredients:

· 4 cups of homemade vegetable stock or broth

· 1 tablespoon of coconut oil

· 1 cup of tomato concasse

- 1 cup diced white onion
- 2 teaspoons of minced garlic
- 1 ½ cups canned navy beans, drained
- 1 ½ cups wild rice, rinsed and drained
- 2 teaspoons of mixed Italian herbs
- Real salt and black pepper, to taste
- ½ cup coconut cream
- 2 tablespoons of maca root powder
- 1 cup packed fresh kale leaves, roughly chopped
- 1 stem of green onions, chopped

Directions:

1. In a large heavy bottomed stock pot, apply medium-high heat and add the ghee or oil. Sauté the onion, garlic and tomato for about 3 to 4 minutes, or until soft and fragrant.

2. Add in the stock, beans, rice and Italian herbs, cover the pot and cook until it

reaches to a boil. Reduce to low heat, briefly stir the ingredients and cover the pot. Simmer for about 40 to 50 minutes or until the rice and beans are soft and cooked through.

3. While simmering the soup, dissolve the maca root in a bowl with ¼ cup stock and set aside.

4. When the soup is ready, pour in the coconut cream and maca mixture and season to taste with salt and black pepper. Add in the kale and cook until lightly wilted. Remove from heat and adjust seasoning if desired.

5. Portion into individual serving bowls, top with green onions and serve warm.

Broccoli and Fava Salad

Preparation time: 10 minutes

Cooking time: 10 minutes

Serves: 4

Ingredients:

- 2 cups of boiled fava beans

- 1 cup of shelled green pea, boiled and drained

- 2 cups of detached broccoli florets, blanched

- 1 medium red sweet pepper, seeded and sliced into thin strips

- 1 small white onion, thinly sliced

- ½ teaspoon mixed Italian herbs

- Real salt and black pepper, to taste

- 1 teaspoon of toasted sesame seeds, for serving

- 1 teaspoon of chopped fresh parsley, for serving

For the Salad Dressing:
- 1 organic lemon, juiced

- ¼ cup of tahini sauce

- 1 teaspoon of agave nectar

- 1 teaspoon of crushed red pepper flakes

Directions:

1. Blanch the broccoli in a pot with boiling water for about 1 to 2 minutes. Remove form pot, transfer to a bowl with ice bath to stop further cooking. Drain, transfer to a large bowl and set aside.

2. In a small mixing bowl, add all salad dressing ingredients and stir until well combined. Set aside.

3. In the large bowl with the broccoli, add in the fava beans, green peas, sweet pepper, onion and Italian herbs. Season to taste with salt and pepper and pour in the salad dressing.

4. Gently toss to evenly coat the vegetables with the dressing mixture and portion into individual serving bowls.

5. Top with sesame seeds and parsley, chill before serving or serve immediately

Spicy Grilled Hemp Fu with Mixed Bean Salad

Preparation time: 15 minutes

Cooking time: 10 to 15 minutes

Serves: 4 to 6

Ingredients:

- 8 ounces pressed and drained Hemp or soy tofu, cut into 4 equal portions

- 1 medium white onions, quartered

- 1 sweet potato, quartered

- 1 large sweet pepper, quartered

For the Marinade:
- 1 tablespoon of tomato paste

- 1 tablespoon of raw coconut aminos

- 1 teaspoon extra-virgin olive oil

- 1 teaspoon liquid stevia or 1 tablespoon agave nectar

- 1 tablespoon prepared mustard

- ½ teaspoon garlic powder

- 2 tablespoons of Sriracha sauce

- 1 teaspoon of crushed red pepper flakes

- Salt and black pepper, to taste
-

Directions:

1. Mix all ingredients for the marinade and stir until well combined. Add the Hemp Fu and toss to evenly coat with the marinade mixture. Let it stand for at least 1 hour before grilling and soak two wooden skewers in water.

2. While marinating the Hemp tofu, preheat grill to high and lightly brush the grids with oil.

3. After marinating the Hemp tofu, drain skewers and wipe with paper towels.

4. Thread the onion, a slice of Hemp tofu, a quarter of sweet potato, and a slice of sweet pepper. Repeat the order of threading with the remaining ingredients.

5. Reduce the grill heat to medium and grill the vegetables and Hemp tofu for about 8 to 10 minutes while turning occasionally to cook evenly on all sides.

6. While grilling, regularly brush with remaining marinade and discard the skewers from the grilled Hemp tofu.

7. Let it rest for about 5 minutes before serving placed in a serving platter.

Edamame-Quinoa Kale Salad

Preparation time: 15 minutes

Cooking time: 10 to 15 minutes

Serves: 4 to 6

Ingredients:

For the Salad:
- 2 cups sprouted or boiled quinoa

- 1 ½ cups of boiled edamame beans

- 3 cups loosely packed fresh kale leaves, chopped

- 1 cup quartered cherry tomatoes

- 2 shallots, thinly sliced

- 1 cup of diced fresh ripe mango

- 1 cup of diced fresh ripe avocado
- 2 tablespoons chopped, dry roasted almonds

For the Lemon Vinaigrette:
- 2 tablespoons flaxseed or olive oil
- 1 organic lemon, juiced
- ½ teaspoon of minced garlic
- 1 teaspoon of raw honey or agave nectar
- 1 teaspoon of finely minced fresh basil leaves
- Pink Himalayan salt or Real salt and black pepper, to taste

For the Topping:
- 2 tablespoons of dried mixed berry
- 2 tablespoons of dried mixed nuts
- 2 tablespoons of minced fresh parsley leaves

Directions:

1. Mix all ingredients for the vinaigrette in a medium bowl and whisk until smooth and well incorporated.

2. Add all salad ingredients in a large mixing bowl. Drizzle with lemon vinaigrette and gently toss to evenly coat the salad ingredients with vinaigrette. Season with salt and black pepper and chill for at least 30 minutes before serving.

3. Divide into four serving bowls and serve immediately with topping ingredients.

Fava Green Salad with Quinoa and Avocado Sauce

Preparation time: 15 minutes

Cooking time: N/A minutes

Serves: 4 to 6

Ingredients:

For the salad:
- 2 cups of precooked quinoa

- 2 cup of shelled fresh fava beans

- 1 medium head of lettuce, cored and coarsely chopped

- 1 tablespoon of flax oil

- 2 tablespoons of toasted almonds, chopped

- Real salt and black pepper, to taste

For the Avocado Sauce:
- 1 large ripe avocado, pitted and diced

- 2 organic limes, juiced

- 2 to 3 teaspoons of flax or olive oil

- 1 green jalapeño pepper, seeded and chopped

- 2 tablespoons of minced fresh cilantro leaves

- ½ teaspoon of Italian seasoning mix

- ½ teaspoon coriander powder

Directions:
1. Add all sauce ingredients in food processor or high blender and pulse until

thick and smooth. Transfer into a small bowl and set aside.

2. In a separate large bowl, add all salad ingredients and season to taste with salt and pepper.

3. Serve salad with avocado sauce on a separate sauce bowl.

Avocado Bulgur Green Salad with Fried Hemp Fu

Preparation time: minutes

Cooking time: minutes

Serves:

Ingredients:

For the Salad Dressing:
- ¼ cup roughly chopped fresh cilantro leaves

- 1 medium stem of scallions, chopped

- ½-inch piece of fresh ginger root, minced

- 2 tablespoons of mirin or rice wine

- 2 tablespoons of toasted and crushed pine nuts

- 1 tablespoon of rice wine vinegar

- 1 tablespoon of avocado

- 1 large pinch of salt

For the Avocado Salad:
- 1 cup packed fresh collard greens, torn into pieces

- 1 cup of precooked/boiled bulgur wheat, drained

- 1 ripe avocado, pitted and cut into wedges

- 8 ounces of pressed and drained hemp Fu or soy tofu, cut into 4 slices

- **1**

Directions:

1. Add all dressing ingredients in small bowl and whisk until well combined. Cover and set aside.

2. In a large serving bowl, add all salad ingredients and drizzle half of the salad dressing. Gently toss to combine and chill for at least 2 hours before serving, if desired.

3. Serve salad with the remaining salad dressing in small sauce bowl.

Arugula and Fava Salad with Apricots and Hemp Fu

Preparation time: minutes

Cooking time: minutes

Serves:

Ingredients:

· 12 ounces of fried Hemp Fu slices

· ¼ cup mixed dried berries

· Salt and crushed red pepper flakes, to taste

For the Vinaigrette:

- 2 tablespoons of extra virgin olive oil
- 2 tablespoons white wine vinegar
- 1 large pinch of salt
- 1 tablespoon minced fresh parsley
- 1 small pinch of ground black pepper
- ½ teaspoon dried tarragon leaves

For the Salad:
- 2 cups of shelled fresh fava beans, blanched
- ¼ teaspoon crushed black pepper
- 1 cup packed fresh baby arugula
- ½ medium head of green lettuce, leaves separated
- 1 cup sliced fresh apricots
- ½ cup thinly sliced red onion

Directions:

1. Season the sliced hemp Fu with salt and black pepper, and fry in a skillet with oil for 4 minutes on each side. Blanch the fava

beans in a pot with boiling water for 2 to 3 minutes and drain completely. Place the fried hemp Fu on a plate and the fava beans in a large bowl, set aside.

2. In a small mixing bowl, whisk together the vinegar, salt and a pinch of black pepper. Mix in the oil and whisk until well combined. Set aside.

3. Combine all ingredients for the salad in a large bowl, except for the Hemp Fu. Pour in the vinaigrette and gently toss to evenly coat the salad ingredients. Season to taste with salt and crushed red pepper flakes and briefly toss to combine.

4. Divide into 4 serving bowls, top with fried hemp Fu and serve immediately.

Curried Bulgur and Lima Beans with Squash

Preparation time: minutes

Cooking time: minutes

Serves:

Ingredients:

- 2 cups precooked lima beans
- 2 cups precooked bulgur
- 1 cup cubed butternut squash
- 2 teaspoon minced garlic
- ½ cup of dice red onion
- 1 large red tomato, diced
- 1 tablespoon flaxseed or olive oil
- 1 large pinch of asafetida
- ¼ cup fresh coriander leaves, chopped
- ¼ chili powder
- ¼ teaspoon ground cumin seeds
- ½ teaspoon ground mustard seeds
- ½ teaspoon cumin seeds
- 2 tablespoons of yellow curry paste
- 1 large pinch of ground turmeric
- 3 cups of vegetable stock, or as needed

- 1 cup of coconut cream

- Fleur de sel and black pepper, to taste

Directions:

1. In a large pan or skillet, apply medium-high heat and add the oil. Sauté the onions, garlic and tomatoes for about 3 to 4 minutes, or until soft and tender.

2. Stir in the spices together with the rest of the ingredients. Cook further for about 3 to 4 minutes and pour in just enough stock to cover all ingredients completely.

3. Cook until it reaches to a boil, stir to combine and reduce heat to low. Simmer for about 20 to 25 minutes and season to taste with salt and pepper.

4. When all ingredients are thoroughly cooked and ready to serve, remove the skillet from heat and adjust seasonings if desired.

5. Transfer into a four serving bowl and serve warm.

Fava and Broccoli Salad with Tahini Dressing

Preparation time: 10 minutes

Cooking time: 10 minutes

Serves:

Ingredients:

· 2 cups of precooked or boiled fava beans

· 1 cup of boiled edamame

· 2 cups of detached broccoli florets, blanched

· ½ cup of sliced red sweet pepper

· ¼ cup of dried goji berries

· Salt and black pepper, to taste

· ½ teaspoon of crushed red pepper flakes, for serving

For the Tahini Dressing:
· 3 tablespoons of tahini

· 2 tablespoons of water

· 1 lemon, juiced

- 1 teaspoon minced garlic

- ½ teaspoon of seasoned salt

- 1 teaspoon of raw honey or stevia

Directions:

1. Add all ingredients for the tahini dressing in a blender and pulse until smooth and well incorporated.

2. Place all salad ingredients in a large bowl and season to taste with salt, pepper and red pepper flakes. Drizzle with tahini dressing and gently toss to evenly coat the salad ingredients with the dressing.

3. Divide into 4 serving bowls and serve immediately.

Conclusion

Vegetarian diet provides balanced nutrition to meet the body's nutritional needs. It also contains the best sources of plant-based foods from all major food groups to supply the body with right amounts and types of nutrients that are essential in maintaining optimal health and for proper functioning of the body. Superfoods have long recognized for their anti-aging and immune-boosting properties and can lead to healthy aging and longevity. The other health benefits of the diet include strengthening of the immune system, preventing various health diseases and conditions, enhanced general health status and healthy aging.

Healthy Vegetarian superfood recipes are also added in this book, which are easy to prepare and specially created to provide you with varied and delectable vegetarian recipes.

With a plant-based superfood diet, optimum health is achieved and risks to various health disease and conditions are effectively reduced. Regular consumption of nutrient-dense foods like plant-based superfoods maintain a well-nourished body is maintained, and also kept healthy, strong and disease-free to promote successful aging and longevity.

Part 2

Introduction

I would like to take a moment to say thank you and congratulations for downloading the book, "The Ultimate Vegan Diet Plan for Health, Energy, and Weight Loss!"

Inside this book you will discover how all the benefits of a Vegan diet as it relates your health, energy levels and weight loss. You will also get complete vegan meal plans for the entire day.

Disclaimer: this book has been written for informational purposes only, and is not meant to replace a doctor's prescriptions and advice.

Thanks again for downloading this book, I hope you enjoy it!

Chapter 1: A Brief Vegan History

Being vegetarian dates back to the earliest Indus Valley Civilizations. Intuitively it may even seem longer than that, but not much record exists that can substantiate the notion or the concept. Avoiding meat came about for many reasons, including religious, as well as observations of health benefits. Five thousand years later, somewhere in the mid 19th century a term was coined to identify a group of practitioners who refrained from the consumption of meat. They were, and still are, called Vegetarians.

Vegetarianism was rather an all-encompassing term which remained until the mid-20th century when a Brit named Donald Watson decided to refine the physical manifestation of vegetarianism with a more moral imperative, taking animal rights into account. He realized the public relations and marketing ramifications of not differentiating the implications and set about to derive a new name and settled on the term *Vegan*. It was just the word vegetarian that was truncated to only include the beginning and the end - a symbolic gesture of Watson's. He then went on to establish The Vegan Society, which still stands till this day.

The term Vegan, as common as it is today, was not so prominent when Watson first coined it. In fact, he opened it up to the public to come up with a name. Eventually the name was settled upon and life moved on, but the controversy continued. People just didn't get the idea behind the new differentiations. Veganism was not vegetarianism, it was a lot more than that. It wasn't just about abstaining from meat, it was about not doing harm to animals and the added benefit of protecting the environment.

The fact that you intend to, or are thinking about Veganism says three things. First, you care about what you put in you. Second, you care about how the animals are treated; and third, you care about the planet and the environment as a whole.

Our Environment

The term has been used to death, and just like the way a word loses all meaning after you repeatedly say it, the word Environment has been worn out with overuse. But there is a significant correlation between the prevalence and Veganism and the health of the environment. If you understand the circle of energy, you know all energy comes from the sun. Plants extract this energy directly and when we eat plants (vegetables) we get the energy, in just one step.

By choosing meat instead, it is the animal that needs to consume the vegetation (grass, for instance) then humans, in turn, ingest them. This is a two step process. As you ascend the food chain, you essentially get further from the source of energy. This is less efficient.

One more problem enters the calorie intake cycle as well. With every layer that is introduced there is a higher chance and a higher level of contamination that enters the body. This is above and beyond the issue of cholesterol and fat. Take for instance the mercury in cod fish. The mercury contamination in cod doesn't come from the sun, it comes from the cod's eating habits and habitat characteristics.

Then off course comes the issue that many people are familiar with. The issue that is always discussed in public, which is the ratio of intake at the lower levels in the chain. When you eat meat, there is much wastage in terms of the bones, the hide and all the other inedible parts. A cow for example requires 5 kilos of grain just to get back a kilo of meat. Then add to that, there are greenhouse gasses as well, and you start to see that the utility of devouring a cow starts to make less sense. The methane each cow produces, varies. But it can be estimated that on average each cow releases 65 kilos of methane in flatulence alone, each year. This does not include the methane that's released from cow pies.

So you get the picture, eating farm animals is not healthy for you and it has an effect on the planet.

Our Mind & Body

If that still hasn't aroused your attention, let's try one more issue. Eating an animal is bad enough on so many levels like I've mentioned above. But now look at killing the animal or raising it in inhumane ways. Have you seen how chickens are raised? Have you seen how cows are separated from their calves so that we can get the milk, instead of them? Do you know why veal is primarily from male calves? The reasons for all these will shock you.

Farming, fishing and breeding destroy large areas of land and destroy ocean ecosystems. The artificial environment where fish are raised are incapable of naturally and effectively handle diseases that spread in enclosed environments. To counter this, copious amounts of antibiotics and medications are added to the water and sometimes, the animals are even genetically modified for one thing or another. The prevalence of eating meat has gone so far that breeders and agricultural scientists now tamper with the genetics so that livestock grow faster and bigger.

But pressing these issues may just seem a little extreme, so for that, let's just look at one aspect of Veganism, which is the healthy functioning of the body and the clarity of the mind that comes from consuming foods that are not tainted, chemically and morally.

From a moral perspective, the world, and by world I mean humans, needs a moment of pause to observe the devastation caused by the sheer incredulity of our species, causing harm to the human race and the ecosystem as a whole.

We, as a species, need to realize, that we are all interconnected, whether it is the lush green canopy over the Amazon, to the sands of the Sahara, from the Antarctic in earth's basement to the polar bears in the north, and from the bacteria in the depths of our gut to the algae in the sea, we are all symphonically, and symbiotically connected in a very real way. Harm to any group, imbalance to some, or extinction of one, echoes through life and does reach us. Of that, there is no doubt, and no mistake. To take care of ourselves, we must take care of them too.

One plausible way to approach that is to embrace Veganism. By living Vegan, not only do we get closer to the necessary energy source, we reduce the contaminants entering our bodies. Speaking about contaminants, think about it this way. With the Fukushima Nuclear plant pumping thousands of gallons of contaminated water into the ocean, the fish in the surrounding area become contaminated. While the fish may be one way we get nutrition and calories, it is also a way to introduce radioactive contaminants to our system. That's just one example. What about the chicken farms that shoot up chicks with everything from antidepressants to antibiotics and growth hormones. Traces of that enter our bodies and begin to interact with our mind, body and overall well being. One way to lead a happy life, is to lead a healthy one. One way to lead a healthy life is to rid your body of the toxins found in these meats.

Overall Health

It is a verifiable fact that in today's global condition, the more animal product and byproduct we eat, the more unhealthy we get. There is significant risk of cardiac disease and early onset of cardiac arrest. Chances of high cholesterol increase significantly and directly with the frequency, quantity and quality of the meat that is consumed. It has even been suggested some forms of meat and they way they are prepared could be carcinogenic.

If you look at milk, many people are lactose intolerant. If you understand that cows have a very robust system, and one that is very different from our own, you will realize that cow's milk is not entirely suitable for human consumption. It is not that a person is weak, it is that we are not quadra pedal bovines. We are bipedal hominids. What about that makes us think we should be drinking cows' milk? Much less torturing a cow and her calf to get that milk, then torturing ourselves with a product whose bioavailability of calcium is so low all we are ingesting is milk fat, sugar and water.

Eggs are another problem altogether. Raw eggs present the risk of salmonella, not to mention the high levels of cholesterol. The list goes on, but fortunately, a few days of abstinence and you will instantly see the benefits of ridding your body of most of the effects.

The problem with meat, eggs, milk and all the other meat based products is that they are insidious. You do not see the problems they cause as it happens. The incremental changes are almost imperceptible and eventually they strike when it gets too far. But at that point it is too late.

There are a few issues with the typical Vegan diet. You need to take steps in factoring this into your routine. It's just like any diet, you need to balance it in some way for the intake of essential vitamins and minerals. If you had proper access to the full range of non-animal diets then this wouldn't be too much of an issue. However, typically, since the full array is not always available, beware of the following deficiencies that could crop up.

Let's start with Calcium. Most people, with animal based diets, think they get enough from milk. But that is not entirely true. The bioavailability of calcium in milk is low, compared to soy. Drink more soy milk. Calcium is not contained in most greens and legumes but is abundant in soy. Make sure that is something in your daily diet. Another option is to have a calcium supplement.

Another mineral that is essential in the body, one that is found in low quantities in Vegan diets, is Iodine. Low Iodine results in goiter. If you don't get your iodine from milk, it's going to be a challenge to get it from another source unless you are in the habit of adding seaweed to your diet. There are Iodine tablets you can take or you can add iodized salt to your diet. But seaweed is best.

Another mineral that is a heavy requirement is Iron. Many Vegan foods, including leafy greens and certain kinds of beans, are abundant in iron. However, there are also a number of foods that block the uptake of iron from the diet. This is of special concern to women. Menstruation demands that iron be replenished in the system, and high amounts of iron are required for this every month. Certain foods tend to block the uptake of iron and this complicates matters. Black tea blocks the iron intake in many people. Be aware of these foods if you are not getting enough iron or it's that time of the month.

Because Omega-3 is mostly found in fish oil, like salmon, Vegan diets are severely impacted by this. For Vegans the best way to rectify this is by adding walnuts into their diets.

The biggest problem of all is Vitamin B-12. The level of available B-12 in Vegan dishes, versus what you need is severely a problem. The best way to get this, is to take on a supplement. B12 deficiencies are insidious and present in different ways to different people. It may present as anemia in pre-menopausal women, because of the lack of her ability to absorb iron, or it may present as low blood pressure for men who drink a lot of tea. Either way, rooting out a B12 deficiency is not always an easy thing. The best is to get on a supplement right away.

Chapter 2: The Central Diet for Vegans

Handy Ingredients

You will need tofu, seaweed, bread fresh veggies, olive oil, nuts, balsamic vinegar, potatoes, garlic, salt and pepper. Off course you can load up your pantry with a lot more than this, but this gets you started with the most basic home made sandwiches. If you look at Chapter 8, there is a list of your shopping list. It is only meant to get you started.

Healthy Diets

To get on a healthy diet and increase your inner and outer health as well as boost your energy and lose weight at the same time, you have to know what foods are at your disposal. You've already seen the list in the last chapter of the possible deficiencies that can arise and now you need to know how you can get yourself sorted in a world that caters to processed food that is full of animal byproducts.

The key to getting on it and sticking to it is to get your infrastructure aligned and your habits tuned. The first thing to do is to get a number of ideas for daily meals. One of the biggest stumbling blocks to eating healthy and being Vegan is being unprepared. When one is unprepared it's easy to fall back on to easily available meals like from a fast food burger joint.

For this purpose, I've organized your foods into categories that will help you to getting on track as quickly as possible and staying that way.

The first group of easy to prepare items are delicious and healthy. These are smoothies that you can make for a quick breakfast, or something to pick you up when you're running low on energy. Fruit smoothies are a good way to get calories in a hurry and a way to get your blood sugar up, slowly. Make sure you keep an eye on your glycemic index as well.

If you like chocolate, that's fine, you are more than welcome to get dark chocolate and mix it into your recipes. There are

Vegan versions where there is no milk in the preparations.

The second set of foods that you will need are the solids. This is your chance to load up on breads and carbs. The sandwich section is a great way to have a filling meal that keeps your tummy healthy without inviting poor habits and without the bloated and full aftereffect. Sandwiches help you to get your mastication muscles active and by doing that it helps to get your liver secretions up. Chewing is a habit many people take for granted, however, by increasing your chewing, it pulverizes your food and allows better distribution of your digestive enzymes. It also allows your liver to function better. All that from a sandwich!

In addition to the sandwich, there is the salad. That's the obvious group. But I have a few salads that's going to redefine your world of salads. Most salads are great, just remember how you choose your dressing. Some have eggs, others have cream.

So far, nothing too complicated, you didn't even need to fire up the stove. But there is more to life. I will look at stir fries. Personally, vegetables, especially organic vegetables need a good wash, but they do not need to be cooked too much. The lighter they are fired or baked, more of the enzymes and amino acids remain intact.

Then finally there is the vegetables that you can grill, barbecue, broil and bake. These are the hardy veggies that need a little more work and go great with almost anything you can think off. I like to mix them up a lot too. For instance, the sandwiches I mentioned earlier, well I fill them with stir fries at times, or with grilled veggies too and wash it down with a smoothie.

Ok so let's get down to it.

Smoothies

Smoothies are the easiest things in the world. Just remember don't use milk. Whenever I want to make mine creamy, I add bananas - as fas as I am concerned, that's the secret ingredient to a good smoothie. It takes me less than four minutes to get a smoothie together. The great thing about a smoothie is that it can be made with a number of different basses. I use one of either soy milk, almond milk, cashew milk and rice milk.

I make all the milk at home, but you can just as easily buy them from the store. If you want to make it at home, just make a batch of these and place them in the fridge. The milk will last in the fridge nicely for at least a week. I use organic seeds/nuts and soak them in water. After that's been soaked, I put them in the blender and run them for a few minutes. I strain the resulting blend and separate the liquid from the solids. Just to be certain, I boil the milk and place that in the fridge. The solids in the strainer I keep them aside for use in cookies and cakes, and even bread. All the different milk are made the exact same way.

When I make the smoothie, I just take the milk I have and add different fruit to the mix. If you like it cold and don't want to add ice, keep a bunch of grapes in the freezer. When they freeze, they are like little grape-flavored ice cubes that blend very well. If you want to make it creamy, add ripe bananas to the mix. Once it's done, the smoothie is a great medium to throw in a few things that you need from a nutritional perspective. For instance you can blend your walnuts in or you can even add maple syrup for sweetness, or flax seed for your omega-3. I've even blended alfalfa sprouts, and it's great

Sandwiches

For having a good sit down meal, sandwiches are a great way to fill up on a number of daily essentials. I make my own bread, but that doesn't mean you have to too. There are numerous different kinds of breads that will fit the bill. I make mine with just sourdough, without yeast and I've perfected it so much that the bread has its own distinctive taste. I don't use a bread maker, only because the program that runs the appliance is set for commercial recipes.

Mine is fairly easy. I leave a cup of spelt flour in a two cups of water, covered in a warm room. In two days it will sour and form bubbles. I take that and make my first batch of dough. I leave the dough to rise. Then I pinch a handful, and leave that in the fridge. That's my starter dough. I take the rest of the dough, add sugar and some salt and knead it gently. I let that rise and I bake it. The first few batches are not fantastic, but acceptable. But after that, the starter dough starts to take on flavor. The bread starts to mature into its flavor. There is no yeast and no milk. Just flour, salt, sugar. Now what I also do is put in the almond, soy or cashew grinds from when I make my milk. That makes the bread dense and more flavorful. Nothing wasted, too.

With bread solved, the largest part of my meal is done. It is also easy to get Vegan bread at the stores. But my bread lasts a few days and I am in control over what goes into it. I don't use butter since it's a dairy product but instead I use peanut butter made at home and cashew butter, also made at home.

On top of that I have sprouts that grow in the kitchen. The sprouts are high in... well everything. They are super food and I grow them with little to no effort. You can even put them in smoothies, if you like a little green taste, but they manage to replace a lot of the nutrients that would otherwise have to come from supplements.

Sprouts are easy to grow. You can grow them in batches and it can be accomplished in either a specially designed sprouters which you can get at the store, or you can just do it in a bowl at home. There is no need for soil or any other growing medium, or fertilizers for that matter. All you have to do is purchase sprouting seeds, and soak them in water. Be sure to dispose the water daily, or better yet, twice a day. Rinse out the sprouts and put them back into fresh water. You just have to do this for five to six days. By the second day you will have sprouts and by the fifth day they are large enough for you to eat.

Back to the sandwiches. Sprouts are a great topping for veggie sandwiches, especially alfalfa sprouts, which can be eaten raw. Soybean patties fried, grilled, steamed are a great filling, as are dry seaweed sheets. Simple homemade peanut butter sandwiches are also good. In Chapter 3 there are some Vegan sandwiches which I make myself. Simple, healthy and delicious. It's just to get you started. There is a lot you can do, just be inventive.

There are four things every sandwich needs - the bread, the core, the condiments and the sauce. As long as you get these ingredients that fall into one of each of these categories, your sandwich is going to run out great. For these to happen here is a list of things you are going to need to keep stocked in your pantry and fridge.

Salads

To make a good salad, you need to think outside the bowl (box.) A salad is not a mere platter of vegetables, it is a diverse congress of representatives of al that sprouts, hangs, shoots, seeds and flowers. It is a rainbow of colors and a medley of flavors. Don't get caught up with putting in only what you like, play with the colors and the textures.

Salads can be anything from seeds, to sprouts, to roots, to stems and leaves and fruits. The entire life cycle of a plant is represented in a salad and so are the basic tastes that awaken your tongue. And it doesn't stop there, add stuff that gets your nose into the game as well. Put all this together and see your salad come alive.

Salads are about variety, so put everything in and make them colorful. Add grape juice, or orange juice to your salads.

Grilled Veggies

As the name implies, this is a simple process. Just grill the veggie on a hot skillet. There are a number of ways you can do this. Personally, I do not like the use of cooking oil and since I don't use butter and clarified butter, I am left to fend for myself when it comes to cooking or frying. So here is how I handle it - I make my own cooking oil.

By the way, cooking oils that come from the store are extremely unhealthy and so I make my own. It is simple.

If you like peanut oil, the process is simple. Just take a cup of peanuts and add two tablespoons of water. Put it in the blender and let it rip until the whole thing is a paste. Take this out and put it in the fridge. In 24 hours the oil will float to the surface. Separate the oil from the peanut mix. You can use the ground peanuts for cakes and breads. The oil, you can use to stir fry, and grilling.

You can do the same if you want cashew oil or even coconut oil.

Keep the oil in the fridge because it is pure, and has absolutely no preservatives, they will turn bad if you leave them out.

As far as grilling the vegetables, brush them with oil and sprinkle sea salt. From here there are two schools of thought. You can either get a hot grill and sear the vegetable, or you can use a warm walk and slow cook them. I do both, depending on what I am in the mood for. Sometimes I even expose them to a hot grill without any oil then drizzle oil over them after they're on a plate. Either way, it's easy.

Stir Fried Veggies

Stir fries are a fantastic way to make an impression with a date or just if you are in the mood to get a lot of sizzle going in the kitchen. It's also a great way to add a different genre of flavors to the salads in the earlier section. Everything you can do for a salad, you can do in your stir fries, except now you can add everything from mushrooms to broccoli. There is a stir fry recipe in the next chapter.

Chapter 3: Starter Recipes

Handy Sandwich Recipes

Tofu Burger

Grilled Tofu
Caramelized Onions
Almond Grind Bread, Sliced
Sheets of Seaweed

Roasted Veggie Sandwich

Roasted eggplant
Roasted zucchini
Roasted mushrooms
Grilled tomatoes
(Add Basil, Thai Birds Eye Chili and Crushed Peanuts if you want to give it a Thai Flavor)
Sprouts of your choice
Soy Bread
Drizzled with EVOO and Balsamic Vinegar

Detox Special

Broccoli, Blanched and chopped
Paprika
Fresh Garlic, Crushed
Sea Salt
Toss everything and add sliced grapes

BLT Twist

Crispy tempeh bacon
Avocado slices marinated in Balsamic Vinegar
lettuce and apple slices
Sprouts
cherry tomato slices
Spelt toast (or any toast you like)

Mushroom Burger

Grilled Portobello mushrooms
Caramelized Onions
Sea Salt
Roasted red peppers
Basil
Bread

Sliced Delight

Sliced cucumbers
Sliced tomatoes
Sliced red onion
Sliced Papaya
Sliced Apples
Sprouts
Salt & Pepper
Apple Cider Vinegar

Sourdough read

Handy Stir Fry Recipe

Stir Fried Tofu With Broccoli
To Prepare the Tofu

1 12 ounce firm tofu, cube it
1 tbsp. Worcestershire sauce
1½ Balsamic vinegar
To Prepare the Sauce

1/3 cup Worcestershire sauce
1/2 cup homemade coconut oil
¼ – 1/3 cup water
3 – 3 1/2 tbsp. pure maple syrup
1 – 1½ tbsp. freshly squeezed lemon juice
1 tsp blackstrap molasses
6 large cloves garlic, minced
I inch young ginger, freshly grated
Stir-Fry Mix

½ – 1 tbsp. homemade coconut oil
5 cups broccoli, cut into florets and stalks, trimmed, and sliced in sticks
3 pinches of sea salt or Himalayan Salt
1 tbsp. Water

1 cups red, yellow, and orange bell pepper, sliced

½ – ¾ cup raw cashews

1/2 cup sliced green onions

There are a few steps to this recipe. You need to sizzle the tofu, so rinse it once you get it out of its packaging, then drip dry it so that it doesn't splatter when it hits hot oil. Pour the coconut oil into a skillet or a wok and heat it till it starts to bubble. A good way to know if it's ready is to throw in a slice of shredded ginger and if it sizzles, you're there. Take out the ginger, or it will burn. Discard that one or put it with the other ginger for use later.

Once the oil is hot, place the tofu cubes in the hot oil and allow it to evenly spread across the skillet. Keep tossing it so that it remains off the bottom and cooks rather than burns. If you do it fast, and with a little bit of practice you will, the frying takes just a few minutes. Once the tofu turns crispy on the outside and brown, remove it off the skillet and let it cool close by.

Return the skillet to the heat and add more peanut oil, which will heat up faster this time. Sauté the chopped garlic and the shredded ginger. If you like sauté the shredded ginger first, then remove it, you can use it as a garnish later. Fry the garlic, then add the water. Before the water boils add the Worcestershire sauce and the molasses. Bring this to a boil, it should thicken. Add the lemon juice to this and take it off the heat.

Place the sauce in a bowl. Return the skillet to the flame and add the last batch of coconut oil. warm it, then throw in the broccoli stems first (they take longer to cook) followed by the florets, the bell peppers, and the sliced onions. Once they are all mixed, add water and close for about 30 seconds. Allow the water to evaporate and add the fried tofu to the veggies. Then add the sauce.

Stir everything together, empty it onto a plate, then garnish the plate with the fried ginger.

Chapter 4: Food Groups

Now, I have no intention of turning this book into a recipe book. You don't really need those these days. Just hop on the Internet and you can find the best recipes and ideas for foods. However, there is one thing that I want to highlight about all these recipes and my philosophy on food. Food is an opportunity to energize the body, sharpen the mind and enrich the soul. If evolution had wanted us to just gain energy for daily sustenance, than we would have a way of absorbing direct sunlight. Instead, we have options. So we need to make use of that.

The first thing about Veganism is that we are acknowledging that everything has life and that we have a moral imperative to do right by all that lives. Someone once declared that our body is a temple, and indeed, it should be taken that way. Meat foods these days have been polluted and they are, for all intents and purposes, toxic, in my opinion.

By being Vegan, we have the opportunity to treat our bodies right and we do this by being conscious of what the body needs to function optimally. Here is a simple guide of nutrients and what we need to perform at our peak.

Carbohydrates

The largest part of our intake consists of carbohydrates. It is the key source of energy. The body takes the carbs we feed it, breaks it down to sugars and feeds our cells that use it as energy. Carbs are to humans, what sunlight and carbon dioxide is to plants. For Vegans, carbs can be found in various categories of food. There are loads of healthy carbs in fruits and vegetables, whole grains and legumes. As much as possible, eating any of these whole is better for you than getting the processed version.

Proteins

Proteins are usually associated with meat products and this is usually a concern for Vegans. But that is only myth. There are plenty of proteins in the Vegan world and without getting too caught up with protein counts, just make sure that you are getting about 0.9 grams for every kg of body weight. Most common sources of protein for Vegans include bread, peanuts and peanut butter, soybeans, tofu, broccoli and lentils. However, my favorite source of proteins comes from sprouts, especially alfalfa sprouts.

Fat

Here is a contentious issue. Most people coil when fat is discussed. However, fat is a requirement for the body. It is the form in which our body stores fuel. Fat is one of the most efficient mechanisms of storing fuel because it takes less energy to form, then reconvert, allowing the body to store energy for use at a different point than it is consumed. Don't knock fat. There are other reasons you need it. There are certain vitamins, essential to your body, that are only fat soluble. This means, that without fat, your body will not get some of the vitamins it needs. Vitamins A, D, E and K are examples of fat soluble vitamins. Fat is also a requirement in the metabolism of cholesterol. A good source of fats include mustard seeds, green leafy vegetables, grains and Spirulina. Of the whole lot, my favorite is Spirulina. Spirulina is also a high source of vitamins and proteins. It also has a high iron content.

Vitamin A

Vitamin A is one of the fat soluble vitamins that are an important part of the body's ability to function. A deficiency usually presents symptoms in vision. The thing about Vitamin A is that there are numerous sources and they come from animal products. However, the body can do some level of conversion as long as we consume carotenoids. One of the more common carotenoids is beta-carotene, found in orange carrots. A good source of carotenoids include spinach, carrots, apricots, mangoes and sweet potatoes.

Vitamin C

Vitamin C is an important vitamin that also happens to be water soluble. This is a good thing because that means two things. First, it easily soluble, and second, it's hard to overdose on it as it gets flushed out with water. Vitamin C helps in the growth and repair of tissues, which is especially important when you are coming down with a flu. It helps to heal wounds and scar tissue and also repairs bones and teeth. For Vegans, there is generally no shortage of this vitamin as it is found in many fruits and vegetables. Just remember heat destroys vitamin C, so try not to cook everything.

Vitamin B1

Thiamin is a highly required Vitamin but also one that is found to be highly deficient in many people including Vegans. Most of the Thiamin, or Vitamin B1 is destroyed in modern day food production and storage. A good source of Vitamin B1 is asparagus, which if you can, you should grow in your garden. Thiamin helps to convert carbohydrates to energy. A reduction in Thiamin means the reduction in the way we metabolize carbs leading to lower energy levels and higher weight gain. Good sources besides asparagus include peanuts and beans.

Vitamin B2

Riboflavin, as it is commonly known, is used by the body to aid in energy metabolism and in tissue growth and formation. Most times it is not an issue as one can find it in eggs and meat. However that presents a problem for Vegans. Instead, we can also find sources of B2 in almonds, mushrooms, sesame seeds and spinach. I like my spinach raw. But this presents a problem with possibilities of E.Coli and other bacteria, especially if they are organically grown. So make sure you clean them thoroughly. To do that, one thing you can do, is use clean water, filtered and boiled perhaps, and add 4 tablespoons of salt. Soak your vegetables in this then wash them off. You can do this for other fruits and vegetables too.

Niacin

Niacin is another important element in healthy living. It is also a major factor in natural growth. It comes into play for your skin, hair, eyes and liver and, the most important of all, your nervous system. It is also one of the vitamins that helps in metabolism. To get a steady supply of this, keep fruits in your diet constant and include potatoes and legumes. My favorite source of this are avocados, but you can also get them in portabella mushrooms and shiitake mushrooms as well.

Magnesium

Magnesium is also commonly thought of as a problem for Vegans. It is mistakenly assumed that only meats have the necessary magnesium to supplement daily dietary requirements. Magnesium is a major mineral in energy metabolism and bone development. It is also necessary in the proper development of tissue and damage repair. A good way to remember what has magnesium is to associate it with fiber. Almost everything that has fiber, will give you magnesium. Women are at a higher risk than men in magnesium deficiency.

Zinc

Zinc is primarily responsible for cell function and also is an important factor in the efficiency and functioning of the immune system. For the proper function of cell division, wound repair and also the metabolism of carbohydrates. It is not as rare as it is made out to be. There is plenty of zinc in almonds and leafy veggies. The problem most claim is the absorption and bioavailability of the zinc from plant sources. One way to increase the bioavailability of zinc from almonds is to peel them and soak them for a few hours. The enzyme inhibitors are usually found in the skin and peeling them raises the availability of zinc.

Chapter 5: Colors of the Farm

Let's start with the reds you will find in veggies. Mostly anything that you find with red in it is full of vitamin C, like Red Peppers. One red bell pepper has more Vitamin C than an orange. A cup of strawberries has more than the bell peppers. And you thought that oranges were the best.

Green, ironically, is the color of Iron. Whatever you see that is green, think of it as having high iron content. Spinach, is one of those. It is nice and green and full of iron. Just make sure that you get rid of the stems as they tend to inhibit iron absorption. Peas, which are green, and collard greens as well, and Lima beans are all rich sources of iron. Try to increase your vitamin C intake though, because plant irons are non-heme and without Vitamin C, they can be hard to absorb.

Then, there's blue and purple. Most blue veggies and fruits are rich with antioxidants, especially anthocyanin. Antioxidants help with aging of tissue and that increases the health of the heart and other tissue. Antioxidants also contain cancer-fighting properties. There have been lab-tested, verifiable proof that precancerous cells were reduces by half when the test subject was exposed to purple anthocyanin in eggplant.

Chapter 6: Tasting the Nutrition

There is more to food than meets the eye too. There is the taste that you should take into account. There are five categories of taste you should consider in your daily meal, in varying proportions according to what your body desires.

The fist in the list is sweet. Sweets are ok, as long as they are not high glycemic index carbohydrates. Stay away from processed sugars or bleached ones and look at substituting sugar with maple syrup. You can even put them on popsicle sticks and throw them in the freezer for summertime snacks. Don't deprive yourself from sweet, but do cut out sugar completely. There is a difference. A sweet banana, or peach, is nutritious, sugar is detrimental.

The opposite of sweet is bitter. You need to have this in your diet to. One of the best ones is bitter melon. In some countries, they are called bitter gourd, in some places they are called bitter squash. These bitter melons are fantastic in lowering blood sugar levels and balancing a diabetic's blood sugar swings. Bitter invigorates the body. Try putting a bitter component in your smoothie or shake and contrast it with the sweet of strawberries and you will find there is a range of tastes that open up in between. Dark roast coffees are also another group of bitters that work well in a Vegan Diet.

Then comes the spicy flavors that you should include in your daily diet. Spicy does two things. It is a way to kick endorphins into gear and endorphins get you feeling good. Keep the burn to a palatable level and you will find that not only do you start to feel good later, your metabolism is increased and so is your immune system, that's the second thing. You will find that you can maintain a lower body weight by increasing the amount of chilies in your diet.

Then there is the astringent flavors which you can find in vinegars. The acidity and astringency go hand in hand but not always. Acidity sometimes reflects Vitamin C, but not always, however astringency helps to regulate the body's water retention. It helps with balancing the interstitial fluids and helps with a higher weight loss.

Saltiness is a little controversial. But, again, as with everything there must be moderation. Salt is one of those. Don't artificially neglect salt. But do use the healthy kind. Do not get iodized salt or ones that are made in the lab. Natural sea salt and Himalayan rock salt are your best options to keep saltiness in your food. Sprinkling sea salt in your salad activates some of the tastes and the nutrition. But stay away from nitrates that are used to cure. Most times they are chemically destructive to your body.

Chapter 7: Weight Loss and Diets

Most people totally misunderstand the concept of weight gain, weight loss and healthy living. It's not their fault, really. They, as with all of us, in fact, tend to mold our thinking around expert marketing. We are told that this is bad and that is good and this is necessary and that is not, and so on. It is the same in the fashion industry, just as it is in the food industry.

Processed foods are all the rage and provide poor nutrition and harmful additives in many of the store bought foods. Not only do these foods harm us, they put our children on an almost irreversible trajectory of poor nutrition. It is the poor quality of food, resulting from fast food adoption that has resulted in more than 1 in 3 Americans being obese - not just overweight, but obese. According to the CDC we spend more than $100 billion a year on obesity related diseases. If we think there is no monetary cost to poor eating habits, hopefully we change our minds soon. Heart disease, stroke, type 2 diabetes are just some of the complications that are placed in our path when we chose to walk the unhealthy road of callous eating habits.

Being Vegan is about being healthy. We arrived at this point in our life where we have questioned our dietary habits and realized something was sorely lacking and amiss. Our instincts, our conscience and our reasoning have drawn the conclusion that being Vegan is right for us and now we are on a quest to a healthier life. Congratulations. It is the first step of enlightenment. When you look at all the philosophers and prophets of the past, the one thing they all have in common is that when they first start their journey of enlightenment, they all start with cleaning up what they put in them. You are, apparently, there too.

To this, let me add some of my experience. Weight loss is about feeling good about yourself. It is about stepping up to a higher plane and taking control of your universe around you. Your body will always tell you what it needs, if you are ready to listen to it. It's okay to take something sweet when your body asks for it, the same way it is ok for you to take something bitter when you need it. Balance your intake and take pleasure in the subtleties of the meal rather than the loud tastes demanded by the senses.

When you begin this diet, it will be surprisingly easy and you will feel the mental clarity like you've never felt before. There is an easy meal plan to follow to get you started and I've placed that in the last chapter.

When it comes to weight loss, it is best to change the way you see things.

Weight Loss

Weight gain is a function of energy storage. Fat is how the body stores energy. Think about it this way, at the very basics of it, whatever energy doesn't get used, gets stored. Everything we do requires energy. Even as you sit down and read this book, it is taking energy to do so. Even when you sleep, it takes energy to breathe.

Energy & Calories

When you eat, you take in energy, and when you work you use energy. Ok so that's clear now. Energy is measured in calories. On average, this is the amount of calories you consume, depending on whether you are sedentary most of the time, or you are active. Age, gender, and lifestyle determine the level of calories you burn in a day.

	Sedentary		Active	
Age	**Female**	**Male**	**Female**	**Male**
4-8	1,200	1,400	~1,600	~1,800
9-13	1,600	1,800	~2,000	~2,400
14-18	1,800	2,200	2,400	~3,000
	2,000	2,400	2,400	3,000
19-	1,800	2,200	2,200	2,800-

30	1,600	2,000	2,000-2,200	3,000
31-50				2,400-2,800
51+				

Based on this average caloric consumption, it is easy to determine a mathematical certainty. If we consume more than this, we store the excess. If we consume less, we feel hungry and our body calls up energy that is stored in fat cells to make up the deficit. That's the easy part. But we are not fully there yet.

Besides calories that food gives us, we also derive nutrients. Why do we need nutrients? Think of it this way. When you have a car, the gas you pump into the tank only gets the engine going. Is that sufficient to keep the car working? No. You need engine oil, brake oil, transmission fluid and so many other things just so that other parts of the car can work in harmony. Fuel, like calories, is just one facet of the picture.

Nutrients like vitamins and minerals are needed to facilitate complex mechanisms of the body. Whether it's regeneration, maintenance, or whatever it takes to keep the body going, it is accomplished by the assimilation of nutrients. Take Vitamin C for instance. I mentioned it earlier. Vitamin C boosts your white blood cells' ability to ward off invading cells. If you only ate, but didn't consume Vitamin C, you will have energy to survive, but you would be sick all the time and that would be a lousy way to live.

So eating is not just about calories and energy, it's also an opportunity to stock up on nutrients. But what nutrients should we take? This the beautiful part of the picture. You're body tells you when it needs nutrients. You've heard it before too. You just didn't know it. When you get a hankering for something, its your body's way of telling you there is something in there that it needs. Remember, your body doesn't speak English, or Japanese or Korean, it speaks in chemical and electrical impulses. So what you are going to feel is feelings. "I feel like strawberries" or "I feel like something spicy" or "I am in the mood for Chinese" all these are ways your body communicates the needs it has. Feeling like strawberries could be the need for Vitamin C. See how that works? So taste, color and sights are all part of how your body will communicate its needs.

So, how come you feel hungry after you just had your meal? Is your body malfunctioning? Unlikely. When you get hungry right after a meal, one of the reasons is because you haven't given the body something it needs. One of the reasons, women gain weight around their menstruation, is because they lose lots of blood and the body needs iron to replenish it, along with the other Vitamins like Vitamin B to help in the making of red and white blood cells. If you feel hungry then have a meal and nothing in that meal contains iron, your body is going to come back in a few minutes and tell you that you are hungry again. So when women who need iron, don't get it, they keep eating not knowing why they feel so hungry all the time.

Been there before?

While all this is going on, and you keep feeling hungry and loading up, the calories are mounting and you find that it begins to store up - you gain weight. Why? well because you didn't give the body what it wanted in the first place.

What does all this have to do with being Vegan? If for the last 20 years you've been eating steak, your body gets its iron from the meat. The next time it needs meat, it's going to tell you to have a steak. You are going to have a hankering for some meat. But since you are a newly minted Vegan, you fight the urge. Right? You're going to get into more trouble.

So how do you fix it?

You need to retrain your body and you need to do a lot of thinking till your body starts to understand where it gets its nutrients from. Turning to Veganism is a great thing, but you will need to do it right, so that you go the distance and reap the benefits. When you have an appetite for something that's not acceptable, look up the internet for what nutrients are in that and figure out what your body could be looking for. Before long, if you will get your wires sorted and if you need iron, instead of beef, your body will ask for spinach.

Conclusion

Thank you again for downloading this book!

I hope this book was able to help you understand the amazing benefits of switching to a vegan diet, as well as provide you with easy to follow vegan meal plans.

The next step is to take action and start implementing what you've learned in this book.

About the Author

Chris Ford is author of several cookbooks on Vegan diet. He has written research papers on the topic and currently lives in California.

CPSIA information can be obtained
at www.ICGtesting.com
Printed in the USA
LVHW031041060120
642629LV00006B/782/P